Essential Oils

Ultimate Essential Oils Guide and 89 Powerful Essential Oils Recipes!

(2nd Edition)

How to Use Essential Oils for Aromatherapy and Healthy Living!

not engaging in the rendering of legal, financial, medical or professional advice.

TABLE OF CONTENTS

Introduction 1

Chapter 1: Aromatherapy – An Overview 3

What Is Aromatherapy? 3

Why Aromatherapy? 3

What Are Essential Oils? 4

What Are Carrier Oils? 6

Chapter 2: How To Use Essential Oils? 7

Inhaling The Oil 7

Direct Inhaling 7

Diffusion 7

Use a Humidifier 7

Steam 8

Application of The Oil On Certain Body Parts 8

Direct Application 9

Massage Oil 9

Internal Consumption 9

Responsible Use of Essential Oils 10

Chapter 3: Why Essential Oils? 13

Zero Side Effects 13

Cheap and Readily Available 13

Market Availability 14

Chronic Illness 14

Safe 15

Multiple Benefits 15

Detox 16

Stress Reliever 16

Weight Loss 19

Grapefruit 20

Lemon   20

Peppermint   20

Ginger   20

Preventive Uses   21

Chapter 4: Essential Oils And Health Benefits   **22**

Lavender Oil   22

Peppermint Oil   22

Neroli Oil   22

Tea Tree Oil   23

Rose Oil   23

Lemon Oil   23

Geranium Oil   23

Clove Oil   23

Pine Oil   24

Eucalyptus Oil   24

Sandalwood Oil   24

Cedar Oil   24

Citronella Oil   25

Grapefruit Oil   25

Frankincense oil   25

Fenugreek Oil   25

Chapter 5: Essential Oil Recipes   **26**

Organic Oil Mixture   26

Minty Magic   27

Sandal Oil Mixture   28

Germanium and Bergamot Essential Blend   29

Cedar Wood and Lemon Mixture   30

Headache Mixture   31

Insomnia Relieving Blend   32

Lemon and Clary Sage Mixture   33

Lavender and Rose Bath Salt 34

Relaxing Massage Oil 35

Peppermint and Juniper Oil Blend 36

Herbal Massage Oil 37

Moisturizing Facial Mist 38

Lavender with Peppermint Skin Mist 39

Lavender and Tea Tree Refresher 40

The Passion of Love 41

Hot Oil Treatment with Argan Oil 42

Get Clear Mist 43

Chocoaphro Loved Blend 44

Go Away Cold Rub 45

Hair and Body Massage Oil 46

Sandalwood and Lavender Blend 47

Facial Cream with Rose 48

Refreshing Lavender Bathing Solution 49

Refreshing Sage and Chamomile Facial Mist with Lavender 50

Peppermint Foot Cream 51

Refreshing Herbal Face Mask Scrub Mix 52

Exotic Jasmine and Sandalwood Passion 53

Facial Oil with Germanium 54

Under Eye Cream with Baobab 55

Relaxing Lavender and Bergamot Body Spray 56

Macadamia and Rose Lip Sense 57

Spice and Everything Nice 58

Soothing Chamomile Oil 59

Argan Facial Serum 60

Cool Foot Oil 61

Simple Baobab Oil with Lavender 62

Body Massage Oil with Geranium 63

Baobab Under Eye oil   64

Amyris and Jasmine Massage Oil   65

Feel Fresh Shaving Cream   66

Rosehip with Carrot Seed Facial Oil   68

Tingy Peppermint Oil   69

Calming Facial Cleanser   70

Enchanting Car Perfume   71

Soothing Foot Oil   72

Almond and Vanilla Foot Scrub   73

Clean and Sooth Skin Oil   74

Refreshing and Relaxing Ylang Oil Blend   75

Moisturizing Body Butter with Chocolate and Argan   76

Hydrating Facial Mist   78

Uplifting Blend with Orange and Cedar Essence   79

Spray Me with Love   80

Peppermint Blend Diffuser   81

Relaxing Foot Soak with Lavender and Epsom   82

Heat Pack with Castor Oil   83

Backache Relief   84

Spicy Body Scrub   85

Body Lotion with Eucalyptus Essence   86

Perfume Blend   87

Lemon and Tangerine Blend   88

Tamanu Massage Blend   89

Sauna/Steam Oil with Eucalyptus   90

Rosehip and Lavender Oil   91

Nourishing Oil with Macadamia   92

Body Mist with Coconut Water   93

Facial Cream with Rosehip   94

Soothing Blend   96

Massage Blend   97

Au Passion   98

Vanilla Delight   99

Sage Massage Oil   100

Massage Oil with Sandalwood   101

Lavender Temple Massage Oil   102

Baobab Foot Massage Oil   103

Cooling Mist   104

Breath Deep Chest Rub   105

Joint Ache Blend with Soothing Qualities   106

Passionate Massage Oil   107

Essential Lemongrass Oil for Skin   108

Cleanser Refresher   109

Argan Sugar Scrub   110

Sesame Oil Massager   111

Fatigue Relief Body Mist   112

Instant Oil Massage   113

Steamy Sauna Blend   114

Soothing Lavender Skin Spray   115

Relaxing Foot Soak   116

Musky Perfume Oil   117

Conclusion   **118**

Introduction

Today, in this mechanical world, health is considered as the most precious asset of man. And why is that so? Because it is so hard to come by. A perfectly healthy man is almost nonexistent in reality. Of course, there are certain exceptions to this general rule. But what is the root cause for this scenario? It is our attitude towards our health. Over time, it has changed considerably and the importance that we give our health has dwindled over the years.

Man's perception of health has changed over the years. Our ancestors were healthier and lived for a longer duration owing to their conscious efforts that resonated their importance for health. They regarded health with utmost importance and valued it more than any other form of wealth. With the passage of time, we have neglected our health amidst our other priorities and today we spend most of our time in rectifying the damage we had inflicted upon our health.

How can you get back to the phase of everlasting health? Can the former glory be restored to humanity by natural means instead of these pharmaceutical drugs that come with tall claims? It is entirely possible to have a perfectly healthy life, the natural way with the help of aromatherapy.

In this essential oils guide, you will find the solutions for many of your health issues and you would be surprised to know how effectively you can manage your health by natural means. You will realize aromatherapy and essential oil uses hold the key to everlasting health by the end of this book.

In the first chapter of this book, I have answered all the preliminary questions concerning aromatherapy which will throw some light on the subject. In the second chapter, I have

1

listed out the various reasons why aromatherapy essential oils should be given a try as opposed to the consumption of pharmaceutical drugs for improving your health. In the third chapter, some of the common essential oil uses along with their medicinal benefits have been highlighted for your reference. In the final chapter, I have listed out certain easy to make essential oil recipes that can help you lead a disease free life.

I hope your lifestyle undergoes a positive change with aromatherapy. Try it out and see the benefits for yourself. Thank you for purchasing this book. I hope you find it interesting.

Chapter 1:
Aromatherapy – An Overview

In this chapter, I have given an overview of what aromatherapy is all about. I have also highlighted the benefits of aromatherapy.

What Is Aromatherapy?

You might be wondering what aromatherapy is! It won't be a surprise if you are hearing this term for the first time. Aromatherapy is the process of using essential oils with a view of improving one's health. Aromatherapy can be used to improve one's mental as well as physical health.

Contrary to popular belief, aromatherapy is not something that was discovered by the modern man. Aromatherapy has been in practice for centuries. Man had discovered the therapeutic uses of essential oils eons ago and started using it to improve his health and beauty from time immemorial.

Why Aromatherapy?

Aromatherapy has multiple benefits. For instance, you can address several issues with the application of one essential oil. Some of the important benefits of aromatherapy are as follows:

- It is proven to relieve stress and is capable of soothing the mind. Aromatherapy can be the best solution if you wish to address stress and anxiety.

- It can help in the reduction of sensation of pain.

- It can help in stabilizing one's sleep cycle and in curing insomnia.

- The digestive capacity of the body is improved significantly.

- Usage of essential oils has a significant impact on the health of our skin. It addresses various skin related issues in one shot and helps you in maintaining the health of your skin.

- Using essential oils can take care of any issues pertaining to your hair care as well. It improves the health of your hair and also helps in resolving any issues pertaining to hair growth.

- Aromatherapy is a good way to improve the immunity of your body.

- Many essential oils exhibit antifungal and antibacterial properties. These oils can be used to treat infections in a more effective way than using ointments available at the chemists.

These are some reasons why you should resort to aromatherapy. As you can see, using essential oils can help you deal with many health issues for which we rely on drugs for a solution. In other words, you can say yes to a healthy the natural way by choosing aromatherapy over drugs.

What Are Essential Oils?

Essential oils are fluids that can be extracted from the different parts of a plant. Essential oils have a lot of medical benefits and can help you take care of your health with less effort.

You might wonder how these essential oils are different from regular oils. One of the striking differences between the two is the viscosity. The high viscosity of regular oils is the reason behind their sticky nature while essential oils are hardly sticky. Essential oils have low viscosity. Another important difference is the aroma associated with these oils. Essential oils possess a distinct aroma while regular oils hardly have any odor associated with them. The third difference between the two is that regular oils are derived from the seeds of a plant while essential oils are derived from the other parts of a plant.

Some examples of essential oils are:

- Tea Tree Oil

- Neroli oil

- Geranium oil

- Sandalwood oil

- Rose oil

- Lavender oil

- Lemon oil

- Eucalyptus oil

- Peppermint oil

- Clove oil

What Are Carrier Oils?

While preparing a mixture of essential oils, to ensure that they blend together, certain oils called carrier oils are used. Some examples of carrier oils are as follows:

- Macadamia nut oil

- Almond oil

- Olive oil

- Jojoba oil

- Walnut oil

- Grapeseed oil

Now that all the preliminary questions pertaining to aromatherapy is answered, let us move on to look at how it is beneficial in taking care of our health in the next chapter.

Chapter 2:
How To Use Essential Oils?

The body always requires essential oils. This does not imply that you can use any amount of this oil. You will have to remember that these oils are corrosive in nature and that they can cause immense amount of harm in your body. This chapter helps you identify the simplest way of ensuring that you are consuming the essential oils that are definitely needed for your body to function with ease.

Inhaling The Oil

This is one of the simplest ways of consuming essential oils. When you inhale the essential oil, you are heightening the senses and also triggering the response that you desire from your body. There are different techniques that you must follow when you are inhaling essential oils.

Direct Inhaling
The first way to inhale is directly. You can simply smell the oil to ensure that you have gained the desired content from the oil.

Diffusion
The second method that you can follow to inhale the oil is through the process of diffusion. Through this process, the oil has become vapor that is floating in the air. Try to use a diffuser that does not heat the content since that affects the constituency of the nutrients that the oil contains.

Use a Humidifier
The next method that you can use is humidification. Buy a humidifier and begin to heat the water. Take a tissue and pour

a few drops of the essential oil on it. Make sure that you are not pouring the oil in the humidifier since the oil will only rise to the top making the vapor useless to breathe. Instead, place the tissue in front of the steam that is escaping.

Steam
Boil a huge vessel filled with water. Add a few drops of oil into the water and cover your head and your nose while you are breathing in the oil. You will need to breathe slowly and deeply to enjoy the rhythm.

Application of The Oil On Certain Body Parts

You will need to ensure that the essential oil is being applied and rubbed as indicated on the back of the box. You have to dilute the oil present by using vegetable oil – either the pure or processed oil. This should be done based on the chart that you are provided. This chart helps you reduce the amount of damage that you may cause to your skin. There are certain places you may apply the essential oil to.

- The forehead

- The temples behind the ears

- The neck

- The crown of the head

- The sole of your feet

- The top of your ankle

There are different techniques that you must follow when you are inhaling essential oils. This section covers the basic and easy techniques that you can use effectively.

Direct Application
This is the simplest method of applying the oil to the area on your body. You can take a few drops of oil and can spread that for two – three minutes.

Massage Oil
The other way to ensure that your body absorbs the oil is through a massage. Drop three – four drops of oil in your palm and rub your palms in a circular motion. If you are directly applying it to your skin, you will have to exert a certain amount of pressure onto the skin. This way you will be able to ensure that the oil is not going to cause any kind of irritation to the skin. You need to remember that essential oils are highly potent and will cause a bad irritation to your skin.

If you find that it is difficult to for you to massage the oil without having an irritation, you can add a spoon of vegetable oil to each essential oil in order to balance the potency.

Internal Consumption

This is the best methods by far since it does not cause any damage in general. However, it is dangerous to consume this internally since the essential oils are highly potent and may affect your body. This section helps you understand how you can ensure that the quantity of the essential oil does not affect your body.

There has been research that has been conducted. This research indicates that there are certain essential oils that are more effective when they have been consumed orally. Only the pure form of these essential oils is proven safe to be consumed orally. They are often used as dietary supplements. The dilution of the oil is dependent on the age of the person. The health constitution of the person is also very important. Read the instructions behind each product before you administer the oils orally.

- Take a capsule and fill it up with the essential oil. Make sure that you wash it down with a lot of water.

- When you drink water or milk during the day, you can ass a few drops of the essential oil, say 1 – 2 drops of it.

- When you are making bread or cooking, make sure that you add a few drops of the oil to the food.

- Drop it directly on your tongue and swallow immediately. You will have to be extremely careful when doing this since essential oils in general are highly potent. You will have to test the oil through the above methods before administering the oil directly on your tongue.

Responsible Use of Essential Oils

Essential oils are highly dangerous to use in general. You need to be able to handle yourself and the oil if you are planning to use them for your body. This sections covers the basic tips that you will need to keep in mind when you are looking at using essential oils.

- Use a drop orifice. This helps you ensure that you are adhering to the correct dosage that has been prescribed by your doctor or other health professionals. If you have an orifice that only reduces the size of the drop, you will be able to ensure that your children or any other child will not be able to consume the oil. They will be administered with the essential oil as and when necessary. But if you find that your child has taken a higher dosage of food, you will have to meet a doctor. But before that, you will need to give your child milk.

- When you have young children at home, it is best if you meet a health professional before you give your child any essential oil.

- When you are going to use new essential oils, test them on a patch of your skin. You can try it anywhere since the sensitivity differs. If you find that your skin has turned bright red or has become hot, you will need to wash it immediately. You will find that water is less effective.

- Try to use a new oil at a time. You can use a blend of oils if that is what you would like to do. Apply a few drops onto your body and then wait for a few minutes. If your skin does not show any adverse reactions you can continue to use that oil.

- There are certain essential oils that may sting your eyes and may also sting at the sensitive areas of your body. If you have used essential oils and begin to touch your contact lenses, you may damage them permanently thereby damaging your eyes. If you find that it was by accident, apply 1 – 2 drops of vegetable oil to your eyes immediately.

- Never put essential oils into your ears!

- If you use pure citrus oils, you may find that the exposure of sun has different effects on your skin.

- Do not apply essential oils to the skin where you have used cosmetics. These cosmetics may take the essential oil deep into your body. This oil may then find itself in your fatty tissue, the bloodstream or your skin.

- Never use essential oils on the area of your skin that has been affected or damaged by chemical burns.

Chapter 3:
Why Essential Oils?

Yes, I had mentioned the benefits of aromatherapy in the previous chapter. If that didn't motivate you to try out aromatherapy, I am sure the many benefits of essential oils listed in this chapter will change your mind. By the end of this chapter, I am sure; you will understand why aromatherapy is much better than the usage of pharmaceutical drugs.

Zero Side Effects

As mentioned earlier, essential oils are derived from the different parts of plants. In other words, they are derived from natural sources. This is precisely why using essential oils has zero side effects. This could be an important factor for you to choose aromatherapy over pharmaceutical drugs. We all know that we stand the risk of over dosage or other side effects when we consume these pills. However, these issues are nonexistent when it comes to the usage of essential oils. On the contrary, regular application of essential oils can actually improve your health. The only thing that has to be borne in mind is that some people are allergic to certain kinds of essential oils. So, ensure that you choose only those oils that you are not allergic towards.

Cheap and Readily Available

We all know how expensive pharmaceutical drugs can be because at the end of the day, these drug manufacturers are driven by profit motives as opposed to the healthcare of the general public. Taking care of your health is a costly affair if you use these drugs. Another drawback of using pharmaceutical drugs is that some of the pills might not be available everywhere.

The quest behind these pills may turn out to be costlier than the drug itself. If you wish to stay healthy in a cost effective fashion, then the appropriate solution for you is aromatherapy. Not only are these essential oils easily available, they are also cheap. Another added advantage is that these essential oils can be extracted at home itself if you have the time and patience. Hence the overall cost spent on essential oils can be reduced considerably this way.

Market Availability

When it comes to pharmaceutical drugs, they can be purchased only from the chemists and only with a prescription. However, these essential oils are available in drug stores as well as in supermarkets. So all you need to do while you are out shopping for groceries is to pick some of the essential oils that you need. If you are not keen on purchasing them, an easy way to ensure that your stock of essential oils is replenished constantly is to grow these plants in your backyard. As mentioned earlier, these oils can be prepared at home. At any point of time, you will never face difficulties in getting your hands on a bottle of essential oil.

Chronic Illness

Often, people who suffer from chronic diseases such as chronic cold or arthritis are prescribed drugs for a longer duration. These drugs are effective in keeping the pain at bay. However, prolonged usage of these drugs can have other serious implications on your health. You cannot avoid these side effects because these drugs have to be taken continuously to improve your health. On the other hand, you can cure the aforesaid chronic illnesses easily by using essential oils. Nothing can work wonders with your arthritis like a good massage using certain kinds of pain relieving essential oils. You can get rid of even the worst of colds by a simple inhalation involving steam and few essential oils. And the best part is prolonged usage of essential oils can actually benefit you in ways that you didn't imagine as opposed to causing damage to your health. Simple research will give you the list of essential oils that can be used in different combinations to cure chronic illness. A detailed explanation of the medicinal uses of certain essential oils is listed out in the next chapter which can be useful to identify those oils which can be used to cure your chronic illness, if any.

Safe

Most of the drugs have to be administered in certain conditions and a specific diet has to be followed for the drug to be effective. If you fail to follow any of the conditions, the drug can prove to be fatal. In other words, the risk factor associated with drugs is higher. You would be relieved to know that essential oils do not come with any tags. They can be used without the fear of over dosage. Similarly some drugs can be consumed only under medical supervision. However, that is not the case with essential oils. They can be used at your own will without any medical supervision.

Multiple Benefits

Drugs are generally manufactured only to address a certain kind of illness or a certain health issue. They seldom have multiple benefits. So if you wish to take care of your health in a holistic fashion, you will have to consume a handful of pills.

On the other hand, most essential oils have multiple benefits. They can be used to address several issues at a single stretch. For instance, sandalwood oil can not only help in relieving headaches but also helps in dealing with obesity. Sandalwood oil is capable of reducing your cravings for sweets and can help you control your appetite. Another interesting fact about essential oils is that, when used with other essential oils in different proportions, they can serve multiple benefits. Application of essential oils also ensures that our body is replenished with certain nutrients. In other words, you are doing damage control as well as prevention of damage with the use of essential oils.

Detox

Our body imbibes toxins from different sources on a daily basis. It can be due to the pollution from the external sources. It can be a result of the increased intake of toxins laden processed foods. Hence, these toxins need to be flushed out from the body regularly. Otherwise, it has a drastic impact on the immune system of our body as well as the functioning of the various vital organs. Application of certain kinds of essential oils can do the trick in detoxifying the body and boosting your immunity.

Stress Reliever

Stress has become an integral part of all our lives today. There are several factors contributing towards stress. We tend to overlook it till it affects our health drastically. Stress is capable of affecting all our vital organs at the same time, which makes it important for us to keep a tab on it. Unfortunately, we have been dealing with stress so far by consuming pills that can serve as an anti-depressant or can reduce anxiety. Though these drugs can be effective, they have other side effects. We tend to take sleeping pills and other sedatives to catch up on our sleep when we are stressed out too much. As we all know, stress is never a onetime thing. This means that the drugs that we are using to tackle stress need to be consumed on a continuous basis which may prove fatal. This can also lead to addiction issues in the days to come.

So how can we deal with stress effectively without damaging our body any further? The answer to this question is essential oils. Essential oils can be used to relax your nerves and is said to have an overall soothing effect. This calm and relaxed mindset is all that is required to keep stress at bay. Moreover, emotions and essential oils go hand in hand. Regular application of essential oils can reduce your mood swings considerably.

The list below provides you with a list of essential oils that you can use to relieve yourself of stress. There are a lot of other oils that can be used. These however are the most common.

- Chamomile: There are two types of Chamomile oils – Roman and German.

- German chamomile oil: This can be used to lower the levels of anger and restlessness. It helps in achieving mental clarity. Regular usage of this oil also helps in bringing about mental stability.

- Roman chamomile oil: This is capable of inducing sleep and can reduce the symptoms of insomnia. This also has a relaxing effect on the nerves.

- Neroli: Neroli oil is an excellent anti- depressant. Apart from relieving anxiety, it also facilitates the balanced secretion of hormones by our endocrine system. Imbalance in hormone secretion is often the reason behind mental instability and mood swings and Neroli oil strives to resolve these issues.

- Rose: Rose oil is capable of acting as an effective stimulating agent. It is capable of stimulating the various functions of the brain. Regular application of this oil can ensure that our productivity is improved and the increased productivity can help in dealing with work related stress.

- Sandalwood: Sandalwood oil is well known for its relaxing properties. It also helps in achieving emotional balance.

- Lavender: Lavender oil is capable of adapting itself to suit the needs of the individual. It can induce sleep and reduce the symptoms of insomnia. It is also capable of dealing with anxiety and relieves headaches. Lavender oil is generally prescribed to induce positive emotions and thoughts in an individual.

- Cedarwood: This oil is widely known for its medical properties. This oil has been tested clinically on numerous occasions. The scientists were able to prove that this oil could be used to help alleviate the suffering of the children suffering from ADD and ADHD. It is however, widely known for containing the properties that help a person calm down easily. This oil should be applied at the point where the neck and the head meet. It has quicker effects of relieving stress.

- Jasmine: This oil is a man's best friend! This oil helps in giving your confidence a boost and gives you a new perspective of the world. This new perception is what gives you the optimistic approach to life. You will find that you have been released from depression if you ever had a bout of depression in life. You will find that you have a chance of getting rid of those terrible headaches. You will be able to fight off insomnia.

Weight Loss

This is one surprising thing is it not? How can oil help in losing weight? Is that the question in your mind? But these oils do not only reduce your weight. They help you lose weight and also leave you with a sense of security. They give you a holistic approach to losing weight. Whenever you want to lose weight, you must not think of having a body that is size zero. You need to think of your health. You will have to change your diet along with your lifestyle to ensure that you can lose weight. You will have to add essential oils too!

You will know that there are quite a few essential oils that have a great impact on your weight loss regime. You will find that they have a great impact on your emotions as well. These oils do not only reduce your weight but also give you a little perspective of yourself. You are able to provide yourself with a positive image of yourself. You will be able to love the way you look. These oils help you connect with your bodies in a way you never have before.

You can use the oils individually, but it is always good to use a blend. The more the merrier, remember? You will have to identify the correct portions of oil required to help aid in weight loss. When you are able to strike that balance, you will be able to find that these oils give you a mental and physical balance! The oils stated below are perfect to help aid in weight loss.

Grapefruit

This oil is the best aid if you are on the path to lose weight. This oil works with the digestive system and tries to reduce the amount of cellulite that is present in your body, it also helps in reducing the sudden urges that you have to eat snacks. It also helps you avoid over eating. This oil helps in the toning of the muscles. It reduces the amount of stress that you may face due to your strict regime. You will be able to boost your self – confidence and also accept yourself in a positive light.

Lemon

This essential oil is the boss of detoxification. Your body has germs in it and will also have certain parasites at times. Your immune system gets rid of all these, but with the lemon essential oil, the system works effectively. You will be able to ensure that the body is full of energy on account of the usage of this oil. This oil also helps you emotionally. You will find that you are able to reduce the negative thoughts that you have about yourself.

Peppermint

If you are on the path to weight loss, you have found your knight in shining armor – Peppermint. This oil is known for its mental and physical effects. You find that you have a new found confidence within you! The emotional outbursts that you used to have never happen anymore. You are no longer depressed in life. You will be able to cure your body of any digestive issues.

Ginger

Ginger is your perfect psychiatrist. If it could talk to you, it could not have done a better job! You find that you have a new found willingness to change the way you think about yourself. You will find yourself empowered and with a certain level of inner strength. This oil helps in improving your digestion and also aiding in the curing of any digestive disorders. The oil is the perfect catalyst for the energy in your body. It helps in sending signals to your digestive system and ensures that the fat is being burnt with ease.

Preventive Uses

Essential oils also have preventive uses apart from their ability to cure certain kinds of ailments. Most of us fall sick when our immunity is down. Certain kinds of essential oils are capable of boosting our immunity. For instance, eucalyptus oil is proven to have improved the immunity of an individual, when applied regularly. When our immune system works perfectly, the question of us falling sick is out of the picture. Hence you do not have to resort to aromatherapy only if you are sick. You can choose aromatherapy essential oils to ensure that you stay healthy, free from any disease, as well.

It is important that we resort to natural means to take care of our health. I am sure that you would have made up your mind to resort to aromatherapy for everlasting health. You would be delighted to know the various uses of certain kinds of essential oils and how it can impact the quality of your life in the next chapter.

Chapter 4:
Essential Oils And Health Benefits

In this chapter, I have highlighted some important essential oils and their uses. These essential oils, as you will see, are capable of improving our health in a holistic fashion.

Lavender Oil

Well known for its skin rejuvenating properties, lavender oil can be used to take care of scars, acne and spots on your skin. With regular application, it helps in adding a glow to your skin by cleansing it. Owing to its soothing effect, lavender oil can also be used to address stress, anxiety as well as your fatigue.

Peppermint Oil

Owing to the increasing junk food culture, all of us face indigestion problems at the snap of a finger. Instead of consuming antacids to take care of the indigestion, you can resolve it easily by using peppermint oil. You can also peppermint oil to get relief from severe headaches and stress.

Neroli Oil

Neroli oil, generated from a citrus fruit, possesses anti-depressant, aphrodisiac and antiseptic properties. Application of this oil can reduce the spots and scars in your skin and can also be used for relieving gas.

Tea Tree Oil

Say no to acne with tea tree oil. It is highly effective in getting rid of acne because of its antibacterial characteristics.

Rose Oil

Rose oil can play an important role in improving the health of our skin. It also possesses properties that of an anti depressant and astringent.

Lemon Oil

This oil can be used to derive the maximum benefits by people who have oily skin. The application of this oil can be used to improve your complexion. It also possesses astringent properties.

Geranium Oil

This is another essential oil that is well suited for oily skin. It can be used on acne prone skin as well. It is capable of tightening the skin by reducing the wrinkles. Application of the Geranium oil can help in dealing with several kinds of cuts and bruises.

Clove Oil

This essential oil is well suited for dry skin. It is well known for possessing sedative properties. It can be the best remedy for your toothache. Even a small amount of the oil can be used to take care of the most severe toothache. Since it is capable of improving the blood circulation in our body, regular application of clove oil can help in increasing your energy levels. It can also be applied to relieve pain.

Pine Oil

Well known for its therapeutic uses, pine oil can also be used as a stimulant and an antimicrobial agent. The aroma of pine oil has a very soothing effect as well and that is the reason why it is used in perfumes.

Eucalyptus Oil

This essential oil is well known for its strong fragrance and distinct flavor. It is generally used as a repellant and an antiseptic. Research has shown that eucalyptus oil can boost the immune system significantly. This oil can also be used to seek relief from headache and common cold.

Sandalwood Oil

This oil can help you in maintaining the health of your skin. Apart from possessing medicinal values, it can be used to relax one's nerves. Regular application can take care of damaged skin and restore your former beauty in no time. An effective cure for scars is sandalwood oil. An important reason why this oil is used in most perfumes is its overpowering fragrance.

Cedar Oil

Apart from its strong and relaxing aroma, cedar oil has other benefits. It can be used as an antiseptic and sedative. It is also known to possess diuretic and antifungal properties.

Citronella Oil

Nothing works as an effective anti-depressant than citronella oil. It can be used as an anti- inflammatory compound and as anti- spasmodic. It is also known to possess diaphoretic and diuretic properties.

Grapefruit Oil

This oil is well known for its anti- oxidant properties. It is also effective in improving the quality of your skin.

Frankincense oil

It is well known for its use as an astringent. Apart from that, it aids the body with the rejuvenation of cells. This regular removal of dead cells and rejuvenation of new cells keeps aging and wrinkles at bay.

Fenugreek Oil

It is well known for its use as an anti- irritant and can be used to cure rashes and burns. It is said to have a soothing effect on the skin. It is well known for its properties as an anti- oxidant as well which helps in delaying aging.

Chapter 5:
Essential Oil Recipes

In this chapter, I have handpicked those essential recipes that can be used to improve the quality of your health in terms of stress relief, improved digestive capacity etc. Help yourselves.

Organic Oil Mixture

Ingredients

- 80 drops of marjoram oil

- 80 drops of basil oil

- 8 drops of thyme essential oil

- 8 drops of oregano oil

- 4 tablespoons of sea salt

Method

1. Clean a dark vial completely and allow it to dry.

2. Pour the ingredients into the vial, one by one.

3. Make sure that all the ingredients are mixed well by shaking the vial nicely.

4. Get rid of your hunger pangs by inhaling this mixture. This mixture is also capable of improving the digestive capacity of our body.

Minty Magic

Ingredients

- 100 drops of peppermint oil
- 8 to 16 drops of ylang ylang essential oil
- 4 tablespoons of sea salt
- 8 to 16 drops of Spearmint oil

Method

1. Clean a dark vial completely and allow it to dry.

2. Pour the ingredients into the vial, one by one.

3. Make sure that all the ingredients are mixed well by shaking the vial nicely.

4. Sniffing this mixture can take care of any indigestion problems that you may be facing.

Sandal Oil Mixture

Ingredients

- 4 to 8 drops of sandalwood essential Oil

- 4 to 8 drops of virgin olive oil

- 2 glasses unsweetened soy milk

- 4 drops of honey

Method

1. Clean a dark vial completely and allow it to dry.

2. Pour the ingredients into the vial, one by one.

3. Make sure that all the ingredients are mixed well by shaking the vial nicely.

4. Whenever you develop a craving for sweets or desserts, consume a portion of this mixture. This should help in suppressing the craving.

Germanium and Bergamot Essential Blend

Ingredients

- 8 to 16 drops of Bergamot essential oil

- 8 to 16 drops of Frankincense essential oil

- 8 to 16 drops of Geranium essential oil

Method

1. Clean a dark vial completely and allow it to dry.

2. Pour the ingredients into the vial, one by one.

3. Make sure that all the ingredients are mixed well by shaking the vial nicely.

4. Inhaling this mixture can relax your nerves and take care of your stress levels.

Cedar Wood and Lemon Mixture

Ingredients

- 4 to 8 drops of almond oil

- 4 to 8 drops of lavender essential oil

- 2 to 4 drops of lemon essential oil

- 8 drops of vanilla essential oil

- 2 to 4 drops of cedar wood essential oil

Method

1. Clean a dark vial completely and allow it to dry.

2. Pour the ingredients into the vial, one by one.

3. Make sure that all the ingredients are mixed well by shaking the vial nicely.

4. Inhaling this mixture can relax your nerves and take care of your stress levels. You can also use this mixture as a balm.

Headache Mixture

Ingredients

- 56 drops of Lavender oil

- 28 drops of Basil oil

- 320 ml of sweet Almond oil

- 28 drops Rosemary oil

Method

1. Clean a dark vial completely and allow it to dry.

2. Pour the ingredients into the vial, one by one.

3. Make sure that all the ingredients are mixed well by shaking the vial nicely.

4. Inhaling this mixture can relax your nerves and take care of your headache. You can also apply this mixture on your forehead to get rid of headaches.

Insomnia Relieving Blend

Ingredients

- 12 drops of Chamomile oil

- A few drops of Lavender oil

- A few drops of Neroli oil

Method

1. Take a bowl and add the oils to it and mix it well.

2. Take some hot water in another small bowl.

3. Add the oils mixture to the bowl containing the hot water.

4. Inhaling the vapors can relax your body and induce sleep. This in turn eliminates the symptoms of insomnia on regular application.

Lemon and Clary Sage Mixture

Ingredients

- 4 to 8 drops of Lemon essential oil

- 16 drops of Clary sage essential oil

- 4 to 8 drops of Lavender essential oil

Method

1. Clean a dark vial completely and allow it to dry.

2. Pour the ingredients into the vial, one by one.

3. Make sure that all the ingredients are mixed well by shaking the vial nicely.

4. Inhaling this mixture can relax your nerves and take care of your stress levels.

Lavender and Rose Bath Salt

Ingredients

- 4 cups of Sea salt

- 20 drops of rose essential oil

- 4 cups of Soda Bicarbonate

- 40 drops of Lavender essential oil

Method

1. Take a small bowl. Add the ingredients to the bowl one by one.

2. Mix all the ingredients well till the consistency of the mixture is that of a fine powder.

3. Store the salt in a clean glass jar.

4. Fill your tub with warm water and some of the salt to it. A bath in this salt infused water can relax your nerves well. You can also say goodbye to your fatigue with this warm bath.

Relaxing Massage Oil

Ingredients

- 28 drops of Sandalwood oil

- 20 drops of Rose oil

- 20 drops of Neroli oil

Method

1. Clean a dark vial completely and allow it to dry.

2. Pour the ingredients into the vial, one by one.

3. Make sure that all the ingredients are mixed well by shaking the vial nicely.

4. A nice massage using this mixture can get rid of your stress. For better results, heat the oil for a few seconds and apply it on your body.

Peppermint and Juniper Oil Blend

Ingredients

- 2 tablespoon jojoba oil

- 6 drops juniper berry essential oil

- 6 drops peppermint essential oil

- 4 tablespoons sweet almond oil

- 6 drops lavandin essential oil

Method

1. Clean a dark vial thoroughly and allow it to dry.

2. Pour the ingredients into the vial, one by one.

3. Shake it well to mix the ingredients thoroughly. Be careful while shaking. Churn the vial between your palms carefully.

4. Store in a cool, dry, and dark place.

5. Use as a massage oil when your muscles get sore for instant relief.

Herbal Massage Oil

Ingredients

- 2 tablespoons grape seed

- 4 tablespoons sweet almond oil

- 6 drops lavender essential oil

- 6 drops eucalyptus essential oil

- 6 drops peppermint essential oil

Method

1. Clean a dark vial thoroughly and allow it to dry.

2. Pour the ingredients into the vial, one by one.

3. Shake it well to mix the ingredients thoroughly. Be careful while shaking. Churn the vial between your palms carefully.

4. Store in a cool, dry, and dark place.

5. Useful to soothe the muscles after a long and tiring day.

Moisturizing Facial Mist

Ingredients

- 8 ounces water

- 50 drops Rose Essentials

- 2teaspoons vegetable glycerin

Method

1. Take a mist bottle and clean it well. Let it dry.

2. Add all the ingredients one by one to the bottle when it has dried.

3. Screw the lid tight and shake the bottle to mix the ingredients well.

4. Mist your face and neck whenever you feel tired or your face feels dried out to feel fresh. The mist is hygroscopic so it will fetch moisture from the atmosphere to hydrate your skin.

Lavender with Peppermint Skin Mist

Ingredients

- 50 drops lavender essential oil

- 25 drops spearmint essential oil

- 25 drops peppermint essential oil

- 1 teaspoon sweet almond oil

- 8 ounces water

Method

1. Take a mist bottle and clean it well. Let it dry.

2. Add all the ingredients one by one to the bottle when it has dried.

3. Screw the lid tight and shake the bottle to mix the ingredients well.

4. Keep in a refrigerator for extra cool effect.

5. Do a spot test and then mist your face lightly to counter the attack of the heat.

Lavender and Tea Tree Refresher

Ingredients

- 7 drops lavender tea tree oil

- 2 teaspoons jojoba oil

Method

1. Clean a dark vial thoroughly and allow it to dry.

2. Pour the ingredients into the vial, one by one.

3. Shake it well to mix the ingredients thoroughly. Be careful while shaking. Churn the vial between your palms carefully.

4. Store in a cool, dry, and dark place. Use it to moisturize your skin. It also has a refreshing effect.

The Passion of Love

Ingredients

- 7 drops orange essential oil

- 80 drops Vanilla Essential oil

- 20 drops rose essential oil

- 4 drops cardamom essential oil

Method

1. Clean a dark vial thoroughly and allow it to dry.

2. Pour the ingredients into the vial, one by one.

3. Shake it well to mix the ingredients thoroughly. Be careful while shaking. Churn the vial between your palms carefully.

4. Store in a cool, dry, and dark place.

5. Mix with a little lotion and massage your lover for an aphrodisiac effect.

Hot Oil Treatment with Argan Oil

Ingredients

- 24 drops rosemary essential oil (Use Lavender Oil for Light hair)

- 4 tablespoons Argan oil

Method

1. Take a glass container and clean it thoroughly. Let it dry.

2. Mix both the oils well in the container.

3. Heat the oil lightly in a water bath.

4. Massage your hair and body with the warm oil and let it get soaked by your skin.

5. Shower after done.

6. This treatment will help to soothe your nerves and calm your senses.

Get Clear Mist

Ingredients

- 24 drops sage essential oil

- 8 ounces water

- 24 drops coriander essential oil

Method

1. Take a mist bottle and clean it well. Let it dry.

2. Add all the ingredients one by one to the bottle when it has dried.

3. Screw the lid tight and shake the bottle to mix the ingredients well.

4. Spray around yourself in the air for an invigorating and uplifting effect.

Chocoaphro Loved Blend

Ingredients

- 4 drops orange essential oil

- 8 ounces cocoa butter

- 30 drops Vanilla Essentials

- 2 drop cardamom essential oil

- 10 drops Rose Essentials

Method

1. Take the butter in a glass bowl and melt it in a microwave or with the help of a double boiler.

2. In a glass bowl, add the butter and all the essential oils and mix well.

3. Pour fast in a wide, airtight glass container.

4. Store in a refrigerator. Warm slightly with the heat of palms before using.

5. Use to massage your lover for an aphrodisiac and invigorating effect.

Go Away Cold Rub

Ingredients

- 2 drop peppermint essential oil

- 4 drops eucalyptus essential oil

- Massage cream, preferably unscented

Method

1. Take some massage cream in a glass bowl.

2. Add the oils from the ingredients to the bowl and massage your chest with it before going to bed.

3. Be sure to finish the mix or it will lose its potency.

4. Can help to reduce your cold and also has a relaxing effect.

Hair and Body Massage Oil

Ingredients

- 6 drops Lavender essential oil

- 2 tablespoons baobab oil

- 2 tablespoons jojoba oil

Method

1. Clean a dark vial thoroughly and allow it to dry.

2. Pour the ingredients into the vial, one by one.

3. Shake it well to mix the ingredients thoroughly. Be careful while shaking. Churn the vial between your palms carefully.

4. Store in a cool, dry, and dark place.

5. Use as a massage oil for a soothing and calming effect.

Sandalwood and Lavender Blend

Ingredients

- 2 tablespoons lavender Essential Oil

- 20 drops Sandalwood Essentials

Method

1. Clean a dark vial thoroughly and allow it to dry.

2. Pour the ingredients into the vial, one by one.

3. Shake it well to mix the ingredients thoroughly. Be careful while shaking. Churn the vial between your palms carefully.

4. Store in a cool, dry, and dark place.

5. Rub around your palms and fingers and inhale it for a calming effect.

Facial Cream with Rose

Ingredients

- 1-ounce beeswax

- 7 ounces jojoba oil

- 6 ounces distilled water

- 40 drops rose essential oil

- 30 drops lavender essential oil

Method

1. Take a double boiler and melt the wax in it.

2. Slowly add the jojoba oil and keep stirring continuously.

3. Add the water to this mixture in a thin stream while stirring continuously with a whisk.

4. Remove from heat after a bit and keep on whisking.

5. Add the essential oils to this mixture drop by drop while mixing continuously.

6. Let the mixture come to the room temperature then store it in an airtight container in the refrigerator.

7. Use for a refreshing and enchanting feeling. It will also help your skin to stay moisturized for a long time.

Refreshing Lavender Bathing Solution

Ingredients

- 8 ounces unscented liquid soap

- 4 drops peppermint essential oil

- 14 drops lavender essential oil

- 24 drops cypress essential oil

Method

1. Clean a dark vial thoroughly and allow it to dry.

2. Pour the ingredients into the vial, one by one.

3. Shake it well to mix the ingredients thoroughly. Be careful while shaking. Churn the vial between your palms carefully.

4. Store in a cool, dry, and dark place.

5. Use whenever you want to feel fresh and relaxed. Can be used with hot as well as cold water.

Refreshing Sage and Chamomile Facial Mist with Lavender

Ingredients

- 8 ounces distilled water

- 8 drops chamomile essential oil

- 20 drops lemon essential oil

- 60 drops lavender essential oil

- 8 drops sage essential oil

Method

1. Take a mist bottle and clean it well. Let it dry.

2. Add all the ingredients one by one to the bottle when it has dried.

3. Screw the lid tight and shake the bottle to mix the ingredients well.

4. Always shake well before use because the oils and water will separate.

5. Spray lightly on face and neck for an instant cooling and invigorating effect.

Peppermint Foot Cream

Ingredients

- 1 ounce beeswax

- 8 ounces sweet almond oil

- 30 drops peppermint essential oil

- 5 ounces warm mint tea

- 30 drops spearmint essential oil

- 150 drops lavender essential oil

Method

1. In a double boiler, add the almond oil and beeswax and mix.

2. Slowly add the warm to the above mixture. Keep on whisking the mixture while doing this.

3. Remove the mixture from heat and immediately put the bowl in a cold-water bath. This will thicken the cream. Do not stop whisking.

4. Add the essential oils drop by drop while whisking continuously.

5. Store in an airtight container in a refrigerator.

6. Use when you feel tired or depressed.

Refreshing Herbal Face Mask Scrub Mix

Ingredients

- 6 tablespoons fresh raw almond meal

- 6 tablespoons cornmeal

- 10 drops bergamot essential oil

- 20 drops lavender essential oil

- 4 tablespoons water

- 6 drops sage essential oil

Method

1. In a bowl, add the corn and almond meal. Toss.

2. Add all the oils one by one to the bowl and mix well.

3. Now slowly add the water and whisk until a creamy paste is formed.

4. Store in an airtight container in refrigerator.

5. Whenever you feel tired, fatigued apply the mask to your face gently in circular motion. Let it dry and then wash with lukewarm water. You will feel calm and relax instantly.

Exotic Jasmine and Sandalwood Passion

Ingredients

- 6 drops jasmine oil

- 6 tablespoons jojoba oil

- 6 drops sandalwood essential oil

- 6 drops lemon essential oil

Method

1. Clean a dark vial thoroughly and allow it to dry.

2. Pour the ingredients into the vial, one by one.

3. Shake it well to mix the ingredients thoroughly. Be careful while shaking. Churn the vial between your palms carefully.

4. Store in a cool, dry, and dark place.

5. Dab lightly on your pulse points to smell in the refreshing aroma throughout the day.

Facial Oil with Germanium

Ingredients

- 6 drops geranium essential oil

- 2-teaspoon Argan oil

- 2 drop vitamin E oil

Method

1. Clean a dark vial thoroughly and allow it to dry.

2. Pour the ingredients into the vial, one by one.

3. Shake it well to mix the ingredients thoroughly. Be careful while shaking. Churn the vial between your palms carefully.

4. Store in a cool, dry, and dark place.

5. Massage your face lightly with this oil twice a day for calming effect.

Under Eye Cream with Baobab

Ingredients

- 2 ounce baobab oil

- 20 drops Rose Essential oil

- 2 ounce jojoba oil

- 4 drops carrot seed essential oil

Method

1. Clean a dark vial thoroughly and allow it to dry.

2. Pour the ingredients into the vial, one by one.

3. Shake it well to mix the ingredients thoroughly. Be careful while shaking. Churn the vial between your palms carefully.

4. Store in a cool, dry, and dark place.

5. Dab lightly under your eyes with a ball of cotton every night before you go to bed. This will not only keep your eyes healthy but will also help you to sleep.

Relaxing Lavender and Bergamot Body Spray

Ingredients

- 45 drops bergamot essential oil

- 45 drops lavender essential oil

- 2 drop juniper berry essential oil

- 8 drops patchouli essential oil

Method

1. Take a mist bottle and clean it well. Let it dry.

2. Add all the ingredients one by one to the bottle when it has dried.

3. Screw the lid tight and shake the bottle to mix the ingredients well.

4. Mist your face lightly with this solution twice a day for a soothing effect.

Macadamia and Rose Lip Sense

Ingredients

- 4 tablespoons jojoba oil

- 25 drops rose essential oil

- 4 tablespoons macadamia oil

- 1/2 teaspoon Vitamin E oil

Method

1. Clean a dark vial thoroughly and allow it to dry.

2. Pour the ingredients into the vial, one by one.

3. Shake it well to mix the ingredients thoroughly. Be careful while shaking. Churn the vial between your palms carefully.

4. Store in a cool, dry, and dark place.

5. Dab lightly on pulse points when feeling fatigued.

Spice and Everything Nice

Ingredients

- 6 drops rose essential oil

- 4 tablespoons unscented massage cream

- 2 drops clove essential oil

- 6 drops Vanilla oil

Method

1. Clean a dark vial thoroughly and allow it to dry.

2. Pour the ingredients into the vial, one by one.

3. Shake it well to mix the ingredients thoroughly. Be careful while shaking. Churn the vial between your palms carefully.

4. Store in a cool, dry, and dark place.

5. Mix with Massage Cream and massage for an aphrodisiac and soothing effect.

Soothing Chamomile Oil

Ingredients

- 2 drops lavender essential oil

- 20 drops German Chamomile oil

Method

1. Clean a dark vial thoroughly and allow it to dry.

2. Pour the ingredients into the vial, one by one.

3. Shake it well to mix the ingredients thoroughly. Be careful while shaking. Churn the vial between your palms carefully.

4. Store in a cool, dry, and dark place.

5. Massage your temple lightly for a calming effect.

Argan Facial Serum

Ingredients

- 10 drops Rose oil

- 2 drops lavender tea tree oil

- 2 teaspoons Argan oil

Method

1. Clean a dark vial thoroughly and allow it to dry.

2. Pour the ingredients into the vial, one by one.

3. Shake it well to mix the ingredients thoroughly. Be careful while shaking. Churn the vial between your palms carefully.

4. Store in a cool, dry, and dark place.

5. Massage your face lightly with this oil and let your skin soak it up for an invigorating experience.

Cool Foot Oil

Ingredients

- 2 ounce baobab oil

- 4 drops peppermint essential oil

- 4 drops lemon essential oil

- 4 drops sweet basil oil

Method

1. Clean a dark vial thoroughly and allow it to dry.

2. Pour the ingredients into the vial, one by one.

3. Shake it well to mix the ingredients thoroughly. Be careful while shaking. Churn the vial between your palms carefully.

4. Store in a cool, dry, and dark place.

5. Rub your feet with this oil for a cooling effect.

Simple Baobab Oil with Lavender

Ingredients

- 12 drops lavender essential oil

- 2 tablespoon baobab oil

Method

1. Clean a dark vial thoroughly and allow it to dry.

2. Pour the ingredients into the vial, one by one.

3. Shake it well to mix the ingredients thoroughly. Be careful while shaking. Churn the vial between your palms carefully.

4. Store in a cool, dry, and dark place.

5. Massage your temple with this solution for a calming effect.

Body Massage Oil with Geranium

Ingredients

- 12 drops lavender essential oil

- 2 ounce Grapeseed oil

- 12 drops geranium essential oil

Method

1. Clean a dark vial thoroughly and allow it to dry.

2. Pour the ingredients into the vial, one by one.

3. Shake it well to mix the ingredients thoroughly. Be careful while shaking. Churn the vial between your palms carefully.

4. Store in a cool, dry, and dark place.

5. Use as a body Massage oil for soothing the aching muscles.

Baobab Under Eye oil

Ingredients

- 6 teaspoons jojoba oil

- 10 drops Neroli oil

- 6 teaspoons baobab oil

- 10drops carrot seed essential oil

Method

1. In a small saucepan heat the baobab and the jojoba oils over low heat.

2. Remove from stovetop and stir.

3. After a few minutes add the other essential oils.

4. Store in a cool and dry place.

5. Apply gently around the eyes for a soothing effect.

Amyris and Jasmine Massage Oil

Ingredients

- 10 drops Amyris essential oil

- 2 drops Mandarin orange essential oil

- 6 drops jasmine absolute essential

- 6 tablespoons Sweet Almond Oil

Method

1. Clean a dark vial thoroughly and allow it to dry.

2. Pour the ingredients into the vial, one by one.

3. Shake it well to mix the ingredients thoroughly. Be careful while shaking. Churn the vial between your palms carefully.

4. Store in a cool, dry, and dark place.

5. Use as a body Massage oil for soothing effect.

Feel Fresh Shaving Cream

Ingredients

- 2 teaspoon baking soda

- 3 cups distilled water

- 4 tablespoons tamanu oil

- 24 drops lavender essential oil

- 4 tablespoons sweet almond oil

- 1 cup aloe Vera gel

- 4 tablespoons cocoa butter

- 2 tablespoons castile soap

Method

1. In a double boiler heat the almond oil and tamanu oil with butter on low heat.

2. Stir continuously until the mixture clears.

3. Pour the clear mixture in a large bowl and keep it aside.

4. Take a saucepan and heat water in it on low heat.

5. Add the soap and baking soda to this and stir continent until both the things get dissolved in the water.

6. Add aloe to the water and stir continuously.

7. Put the soap mix in the large bowl with oil and stir.

8. Add all the essential oils to the bowl and stir well.

9. Use a hand blender to blend the above mixture thoroughly.

10. Store in an airtight container.

11. Use for shaving, it'll calm your senses and will keep you fresh throughout the day.

Rosehip with Carrot Seed Facial Oil

Ingredients

- 12 drops geranium essential oil

- 12 drops carrot seed essential oil

- 1-ounce rosehip oil

- 1-ounce Grapeseed oil

- 12 drops Rose Essentials Oil

Method

1. Clean a dark vial thoroughly and allow it to dry.

2. Pour the ingredients into the vial, one by one.

3. Shake it well to mix the ingredients thoroughly. Be careful while shaking. Churn the vial between your palms carefully.

4. Store in a cool, dry, and dark place.

5. Put a dropper cap on the bottle and drop a few drops on your fingertips to massage lightly.

Tingy Peppermint Oil

Ingredients

- 28 drops peppermint essential oil

- 2 ounce sweet almond oil

Method

1. Clean a dark vial thoroughly and allow it to dry.

2. Pour the ingredients into the vial, one by one.

3. Shake it well to mix the ingredients thoroughly. Be careful while shaking. Churn the vial between your palms carefully.

4. Store in a cool, dry, and dark place.

5. Use as a lip balm at night to soothen your lips.

Calming Facial Cleanser

Ingredients

- 7 drops lavender tea tree essential oil
- 1/2 ounce bentonite clay powder
- 1 1/2 tablespoons water

Method

1. In a bowl, mix all the ingredients well.

2. Wash your face with a mild soap and apply this paste.

3. Let it dry for 30 minutes.

4. Rinse with lukewarm water and dab with a towel to dry your skin.

5. It has a purifying and relaxing effect.

Enchanting Car Perfume

Ingredients

- 12 drops lavender essential oil

- 4 drops peppermint essential oil

- 4 ounces distilled water

- 4 drops sage essential oil

- 4 drops geranium essential oil

Method

1. Clean a dark spray bottle thoroughly and allow it to dry.

2. Pour the ingredients into the vial, one by one.

3. Shake it well to mix the ingredients thoroughly. Be careful while shaking. Churn the bottle between your palms carefully.

4. Store in a cool, dry, and dark place.

5. Spray your car indoors lightly to freshen your car and your mood.

Soothing Foot Oil

Ingredients

- 2 ounces tamanu oil

- 8 drops sandalwood essential oil

- 8 drops tea tree essential oil

- 8 drops peppermint essential oil

Method

1. Clean a dark vial thoroughly and allow it to dry.

2. Pour the ingredients into the vial, one by one.

3. Shake it well to mix the ingredients thoroughly. Be careful while shaking. Churn the vial between your palms carefully.

4. Store in a cool, dry, and dark place.

5. Massage your feet lightly with the oil at night for a deep sleep.

Almond and Vanilla Foot Scrub

Ingredients

- ½ cup virgin coconut oil

- 1 teaspoon Vanilla Essential oil

- 1 cup whole almonds

- 1 cup almond oil

- 1 cup unrefined granulated sugar

Method

1. In a bowl add the coconut oil and the almond oil and then melt the oil in a hot water bath.

2. Crush almonds lightly in a mortar and pestle. The almonds should form a fine yet coarse powder.

3. In a bowl, add the oils and the almonds.

4. Add the vanilla oil to the above mixture.

5. Mix well and store in an airtight jar in a cool and dry place.

6. Clean your feet and gently rub some of the scrub on them until the oil is soaked in. rinse with lukewarm water and dab with a clean towel.

Clean and Sooth Skin Oil

Ingredients

- 3 drops carrot seed essential oil

- 9 drops rose essential oil

- 3 drops German Chamomile Essential oil

Method

1. Clean a dark vial thoroughly and allow it to dry.

2. Pour the ingredients into the vial, one by one.

3. Shake it well to mix the ingredients thoroughly. Be careful while shaking. Churn the vial between your palms carefully.

4. Store in a cool, dry, and dark place.

5. Take a few drops of the concoction and massage your skin lightly especially concentrating on the dry patches.

Refreshing and Relaxing Ylang Oil Blend

Ingredients

- 25 drops ylang ylang essential oil

- 45 drops bergamot essential oil

- 50 drops mandarin orange essential oil

Method

1. Clean a dark vial thoroughly and allow it to dry.

2. Pour the ingredients into the vial, one by one.

3. Shake it well to mix the ingredients thoroughly. Be careful while shaking. Churn the vial between your palms carefully.

4. Store in a cool, dry, and dark place.

5. Put a few drops of this mixture in an aromatherapy lamp and relax.

Moisturizing Body Butter with Chocolate and Argan

Ingredients

- 1 teaspoon sweet orange essential oil

- 6 ounces cocoa butter

- 3 teaspoons Argan oil

- 1 teaspoon Neroli oil

- 1 cup coconut oil

- 3tablespoons vitamin E oil

Method

1. Heat the cocoa butter and the coconut oil in a double boiler till it melts.

2. Add the Argan oil to the above mixture slowly.

3. Remove it from the heat and then add the vitamin oil while stirring continuously.

4. Keep aside for a bit until the oil starts to solidify.

5. Whip again.

6. Put the mixture in a mixing bowl and blend with a hand blender.

7. While blending add the Neroli oil and the orange oil.

8. Stop when a light and fluffy butter is formed. Put this into airtight jar and store in a cool and dry place.

9. Use for a moisturizing and soothing effect.

Hydrating Facial Mist

Ingredients

- 7 ounces water

- 6 drops carrot seed essential oil

- 30 drops baobab oil

- 15 drops geranium essential oil

- 20 drops lavender essential oil

Method

1. Clean a dark mist bottler thoroughly and allow it to dry.

2. Pour the ingredients into the bottle, one by one.

3. Shake it well to mix the ingredients thoroughly. Be careful while shaking. Churn the bottle between your palms carefully.

4. Store in a cool, dry, and dark place.

5. Spray your face and neck area lightly when to relieve stress.

Uplifting Blend with Orange and Cedar Essence

Ingredients

- 20 drops cedar essential oil

- 60 drops juniper berry essential oil

- 50 drops bergamot orange essential oil

- 40 drops sandalwood essential oil

- 30 drops fir needle essential oil

Method

1. Clean a dark vial thoroughly and allow it to dry.

2. Pour the ingredients into the vial, one by one.

3. Shake it well to mix the ingredients thoroughly. Be careful while shaking. Churn the vial between your palms carefully.

4. Store in a cool, dry, and dark place.

5. Dab lightly on pressure points when you feel tired or exhausted.

Spray Me with Love

Ingredients

- 10 drops ylang ylang essential oil

- 1 drop clove bud essential oil

- 5 drops rose absolute essential oil

Method

1. Clean a dark vial thoroughly and allow it to dry.

2. Pour the ingredients into the vial, one by one.

3. Shake it well to mix the ingredients thoroughly. Be careful while shaking. Churn the vial between your palms carefully.

4. Store in a cool, dry, and dark place.

5. Shake well before using.

6. Dab lightly on the pressure points for a refreshing effect.

Peppermint Blend Diffuser

Ingredients

- 4 drops patchouli essential oil

- 8 drops peppermint essential oil

- 6 tablespoons water

- 12 drops sweet orange essential oil

Method

1. In a bowl add some water and place a candle at the center.

2. Add essential oils to the water.

3. Light the candle and diffuse for half an hour for a relaxing effect.

Relaxing Foot Soak with Lavender and Epsom

Ingredients

- 4 tablespoons sea salt

- 40 drops lavender essential oil

- 4 tablespoons Epsom salts

- 2 tablespoons baking soda

- 10 drops spearmint essential oil

- 10 drops peppermint essential oil

Method

1. Mix the dry ingredients in a bowl.

2. Slowly add the essential oils to the bowl.

3. Transfer the mix to an airtight container.

4. To use put a tablespoon of the mixture in a bucket full of hot water and soak your feet for a relaxing effect.

Heat Pack with Castor Oil

Ingredients

- 4 drops peppermint essential oil

- 2 tablespoons castor oil

- 2 drops lavender essential oil

- 2 drops eucalyptus essential oil

Method

1. In a bowl, add all the oils and mix.

2. Lightly soak some towels with this mixture and cover a heat pad with these towels.

3. Use this as a heat pad for a soothing effect.

Backache Relief

Ingredients

- 20 drops German Chamomile oil

- 2 drops clove bud essential oil

- 4 drops wintergreen essential oil

- 6 drops lavender essential oil

Method

1. Clean a dark vial thoroughly and allow it to dry.

2. Pour the ingredients into the vial, one by one.

3. Shake it well to mix the ingredients thoroughly. Be careful while shaking. Churn the vial between your palms carefully.

4. Store in a cool, dry, and dark place.

5. Apply to the sore muscles and massage them well.

Spicy Body Scrub

Ingredients

- 2 tablespoons Grapeseed oil
- 3 tablespoons sugar
- 2 tablespoons jojoba oil
- 6 drops peppermint essential oil
- 15 drops lime essential oil

Method

1. Clean a dark container thoroughly and allow it to dry.
2. Pour the ingredients into the container, one by one.
3. Shake it well to mix the ingredients thoroughly. Be careful while shaking.
4. Store in a cool, dry, and dark place.
5. Use it while showering or bathing for a rejuvenating effect.

Body Lotion with Eucalyptus Essence

Ingredients

- 2 ounces beeswax

- 2 cups apricot kernel oil

- 6 teaspoons lemon eucalyptus essential oil

- 2 cups lukewarm green tea

- 2 teaspoons lavender essential oil

- 50 drops geranium essential oil

- 70 drops grapefruit essential oil

Method

1. In a double boiler melt beeswax and add apricot oil to it. Stir continuously.

2. Remove from heat and keep aside for a bit.

3. In a blender add the green tea and a pinch of Borax.

4. Add the lukewarm wax mix to the blender and blend it.

5. While blending add the essential oils in a thin stream.

6. Blend until the mixture gets creamy.

7. Store in an airtight jar.

8. Use the lotion as a moisturizer especially when you are feeling low.

Perfume Blend

Ingredients

- 12 drops bergamot essential oil

- 6 drops sandalwood essential oil

- 4 drops rose absolute essential oil

- 10 drops Vanilla oil

- 5 drops jasmine essential oil

- ½ fluid ounce almond oil

Method

1. Clean a dark vial thoroughly and allow it to dry.

2. Pour the ingredients into the vial, one by one.

3. Shake it well to mix the ingredients thoroughly. Be careful while shaking. Churn the vial between your palms carefully.

4. Store in a cool, dry, and dark place.

5. Dab lightly at pulse points.

Lemon and Tangerine Blend

Ingredients

- 40 drops lemon essential oil

- 70 drops lavender essential oil

- 50 drops Neroli essential oil

- 40 drops tangerine essential oil

Method

1. Clean a dark vial thoroughly and allow it to dry.

2. Pour the ingredients into the vial, one by one.

3. Shake it well to mix the ingredients thoroughly. Be careful while shaking. Churn the vial between your palms carefully.

4. Store in a cool, dry, and dark place.

5. Dab your handkerchief lightly with the oil whenever you feel dejected.

Tamanu Massage Blend

Ingredients

- 40 drops Helichrysum oil
- 2 ounce sweet almond oil
- 24 drops lemon essential oil
- 40 drops German Chamomile Oil
- 4 ounces tamanu oil

Method

1. Clean a dark vial thoroughly and allow it to dry.

2. Pour the ingredients into the vial, one by one.

3. Shake it well to mix the ingredients thoroughly. Be careful while shaking. Churn the vial between your palms carefully.

4. Store in a cool, dry, and dark place.

5. Use this oil to massage your head in the case of headache.

Sauna/Steam Oil with Eucalyptus

Ingredients

- 2 drops Lavender oil

- 1 to 2 drops eucalyptus essential oil

Method

1. Clean a dark vial thoroughly and allow it to dry.

2. Pour the ingredients into the vial, one by one.

3. Shake it well to mix the ingredients thoroughly. Be careful while shaking. Churn the vial between your palms carefully.

4. Store in a cool, dry, and dark place.

5. Pour a few drops in an electric steamer or in a large bowl filled with boiling water.

6. Use this steam to clean your pores and to sooth your nerves.

Rosehip and Lavender Oil

Ingredients

- 8 ounces water

- 2 teaspoon rosehip oil

- 8 drops rose essential oil

- 80 drops lavender essential oil

Method

1. Clean a dark spray bottle thoroughly and allow it to dry.

2. Pour the ingredients into the bottle, one by one.

3. Shake it well to mix the ingredients thoroughly. Be careful while shaking. Churn the bottle between your palms carefully.

4. Store in a cool, dry, and dark place.

5. Spray your face and neck lightly throughout the day when you feel tired or fatigued.

Nourishing Oil with Macadamia

Ingredients

- 1 ounce jojoba oil

- 60 drops Rose oil

- 8 ounces macadamia oil

- 60 drops carrot seed essential oil

Method

1. Clean a dark vial thoroughly and allow it to dry.

2. Pour the ingredients into the vial, one by one.

3. Shake it well to mix the ingredients thoroughly. Be careful while shaking. Churn the vial between your palms carefully.

4. Store in a cool, dry, and dark place.

5. Use as a night cleanser to clean your face. It also has a calming effect due to the jojoba oil

Body Mist with Coconut Water

Ingredients

- 16 drops patchouli essential oil

- 2 ounce aloe juice

- 16 drops lavender essential oil

- 2 ounces coconut water

- 16 drops lemon eucalyptus essential oil

Method

1. Clean a dark spray bottler thoroughly and allow it to dry.

2. Pour the ingredients into the bottle, one by one.

3. Shake it well to mix the ingredients thoroughly. Be careful while shaking. Churn the bottle between your palms carefully.

4. Store in a cool, dry, and dark place.

5. Spray yourself lightly throughout the day when you feel tired.

Facial Cream with Rosehip

Ingredients

- 1ounce beeswax

- 65 drops geranium essential oil

- 3 ounces jojoba oil

- 60 drops carrot seed oil

- 2ounce rosehip oil

- 6 ounces distilled water

- 60 drops lavender essential oil

Method

1. In a double boiler melt, the wax mixed with jojoba and rosehip.

2. Let the wax melt completely

3. Keep aside and let it cool for a bit.

4. Add the essential oils to the bowl while stirring continuously.

5. Heat the coconut water until it becomes lukewarm and then blend in a blender. Add the wax mixture to this and blend again.

6. Blend until it becomes creamy and then store in an airtight container.

7. Keep in a refrigerator.

8. You can use this cream as moisturizer or night cream. It will soothe your skin and will help you to relax.

Soothing Blend

Ingredients

- 2 tablespoon beeswax

- 12 drops lavender essential oil

- 4 tablespoons baobab oil

- 12 drops tea tree essential oil

Method

1 In a double boiler, melt the beeswax.

2 Add the baobab oil to the melting wax little by little while stirring continuously.

3 After a bit remove from heat.

4 Add the essential oils to this mixture while stirring continuously.

5 Keep in an airtight jar in a cool and dry place.

6 Massage your temple in the night for a deep and relaxing sleep.

Massage Blend

Ingredients

- 40 drops German Chamomile oil

- 6 drops lavender essential oil

- 15 drops Roman Chamomile oil

- 2 drop clove essential oil

- 2 drops wintergreen essential oil

- 2 drop allspice essential oil

Method

1   Clean a dark vial thoroughly and allow it to dry.

2   Pour the ingredients into the vial, one by one.

3   Shake it well to mix the ingredients thoroughly. Be careful while shaking. Churn the vial between your palms carefully.

4   Store in a cool, dry, and dark place.

5   Use it as massage oil after heavy work.

Au Passion

Ingredients

- 60 drops rose essential oil

- 6 ounces vodka

Method

1 Clean a dark vial thoroughly and allow it to dry.

2 Pour the ingredients into the vial, one by one.

3 Shake it well to mix the ingredients thoroughly. Be careful while shaking. Churn the vial between your palms carefully.

4 Store in a cool, dry, and dark place for 3 weeks and let it age.

5 Let it chill for a bit after it has aged.

6 Filter using a coffee filter.

7 Chill once again and see if any globules are seen. Filter once again.

8 Repeat until no insoluble oil is seen.

9 Store in a perfume bottler in a dark and cool place.

Vanilla Delight

Ingredients

- 40 drops Vanilla oil

- 4 drops rose essential oil

- 2 drop cardamom essential oil

- 4 drops sweet orange essential oil

Method

1   Clean a dark vial thoroughly and allow it to dry.

2   Pour the ingredients into the vial, one by one.

3   Shake it well to mix the ingredients thoroughly. Be careful while shaking. Churn the vial between your palms carefully.

4   Store in a cool, dry, and dark place.

5   Inhale for an invigorating effect.

Sage Massage Oil

Ingredients

- 2 tablespoon Grapeseed oil

- 2 drops bergamot essential oil

- 2 drops sage essential oil

Method

1   Clean a dark vial thoroughly and allow it to dry.

2   Pour the ingredients into the vial, one by one.

3   Shake it well to mix the ingredients thoroughly. Be careful while shaking. Churn the vial between your palms carefully.

4   Store in a cool, dry, and dark place.

5   Use as a massage oil for a soothing effect.

Massage Oil with Sandalwood

Ingredients

- 24 drops Sandalwood oil

- 4 ounces sweet almond oil

- 24 drops Frankincense oil

- 2 ounce baobab oil

Method

1 Clean a dark vial thoroughly and allow it to dry.

2 Pour the ingredients into the vial, one by one.

3 Shake it well to mix the ingredients thoroughly. Be careful while shaking. Churn the vial between your palms carefully.

4 Store in a cool, dry, and dark place.

5 Can be used for full body massage.

Lavender Temple Massage Oil

Ingredients

- 2 drop lavender essential oil

- 4 drops Frankincense Precious oil

- 2 drop patchouli essential oil

- 2 ounce baobab oil

Method

1 Clean a dark vial thoroughly and allow it to dry.

2 Pour the ingredients into the vial, one by one.

3 Shake it well to mix the ingredients thoroughly. Be careful while shaking. Churn the vial between your palms carefully.

4 Store in a cool, dry, and dark place.

5 Instant relief from headaches.

Baobab Foot Massage Oil

Ingredients

- 2 drops vetiver essential oil

- 2 ounce baobab oil

- 4 drops sweet marjoram essential oil

- 2 drops patchouli essential oil

Method

1   Clean a dark vial thoroughly and allow it to dry.

2   Pour the ingredients into the vial, one by one.

3   Shake it well to mix the ingredients thoroughly. Be careful while shaking. Churn the vial between your palms carefully.

4   Store in a cool, dry, and dark place.

5   Use the oil to massage your feet at night for a relaxing effect.

Cooling Mist

Ingredients

- 6 ounces distilled water

- 8 drops peppermint essential oil

- 2 ounce aloe gel or extract

- 4 drops spearmint essential oil

- 36 drops lavender essential oil

Method

1   Clean a dark spray bottle thoroughly and allow it to dry.

2   Pour the ingredients into the spray bottle, one by one.

3   Shake it well to mix the ingredients thoroughly. Be careful while shaking. Churn the spray bottle between your palms carefully.

4   Store in a cool, dry, and dark place.

5   Spray yourself lightly when you feel tired.

Breath Deep Chest Rub

Ingredients

- 2 tablespoon sweet almond oil

- 10 drops lemon tea tree essential oil

- 6 drops eucalyptus essential oil

- 1 tablespoon castor oil

- 2 drop peppermint

Method

1   Add all the ingredients in a bowl and mix well.

2   Store in an airtight container.

3   Rub your chest lightly with the chest rub for a deep sleep and clear breath.

Joint Ache Blend with Soothing Qualities

Ingredients

- 4 ounces sweet almond oil

- 60 drops Helichrysum oil

- 2 ounce tamanu oil

Method

1   Clean a dark vial thoroughly and allow it to dry.

2   Pour the ingredients into the vial, one by one.

3   Shake it well to mix the ingredients thoroughly. Be careful while shaking. Churn the vial between your palms carefully.

4   Store in a cool, dry, and dark place.

5   Massage your joints lightly to relieve the pain.

Passionate Massage Oil

Ingredients

- 2 tablespoon Grapeseed oil

- 14 drops sandalwood essential oil

- 2 tablespoon sweet almond or apricot kernel oil

- 20 drops rose absolute essential oil

Method

1 Clean a dark vial thoroughly and allow it to dry.

2 Pour the ingredients into the vial, one by one.

3 Shake it well to mix the ingredients thoroughly. Be careful while shaking. Churn the vial between your palms carefully.

4 Store in a cool, dry, and dark place.

5 Massage your partner lightly with this for a sensuous experience.

Essential Lemongrass Oil for Skin

Ingredients

- 12 drops lavender essential oil

- 8 drops lemongrass essential oil

- 2 drop sage essential oil

- 2 ounces distilled water

- 2 drop chamomile essential oil

Method

1   Clean a dark vial thoroughly and allow it to dry.

2   Pour the ingredients into the vial, one by one.

3   Shake it well to mix the ingredients thoroughly. Be careful while shaking. Churn the vial between your palms carefully.

4   Store in a cool, dry, and dark place.

5   Massage the temple for a relaxing effect.

Cleanser Refresher

Ingredients

- 1 ounce jojoba oil

- 60 drops tea tree essential oil

- 6 ounces tamanu oil

- 60 drops geranium essential oil

Method

1 Clean a dark spray bottle thoroughly and allow it to dry.

2 Pour the ingredients into the spray bottle, one by one.

3 Shake it well to mix the ingredients thoroughly. Be careful while shaking. Churn the spray bottle between your palms carefully.

4 Store in a cool, dry, and dark place.

5 Spray your skin lightly whenever you feel fatigued.

Argan Sugar Scrub

Ingredients

- 3 teaspoons Argan oil

- 2 drops lavender essential oil

- 1 teaspoon fine sugar granules

- 3 drops lemon essential oil

Method

1 In a bowl add all the ingredients and mix well.

2 Apply to the skin in a circular motion gently.

3 Rinse with lukewarm water.

4 Has a rejuvenating effect.

Sesame Oil Massager

Ingredients

- 8 drops sandalwood oil

- 2 tablespoons sesame oil

Method

1 Clean a dark vial thoroughly and allow it to dry.

2 Pour the ingredients into the vial, one by one.

3 Shake it well to mix the ingredients thoroughly. Be careful while shaking. Churn the vial between your palms carefully.

4 Store in a cool, dry, and dark place.

5 Massage your scalp for a good night sleep.

Fatigue Relief Body Mist

Ingredients

- 8 ounces water

- 40 drops peppermint essential oil

- 20 drops rosemary essential oil

- 40 drops lemon essential oil

Method

1   Clean a dark spray bottle thoroughly and allow it to dry.

2   Pour the ingredients into the spray bottle one by one.

3   Shake it well to mix the ingredients thoroughly. Be careful while shaking. Churn the spray bottle between your palms carefully.

4   Store in a cool, dry, and dark place.

5   Shake well before every use.

6   Spray generously after working out to conquer fatigue.

Instant Oil Massage

Ingredients

- 1 drop wintergreen essential oil

- 3 ounces coconut oil

- 1 1/2 drops clove essential oil

- 5 drops peppermint essential oil

- 3 drops orange essential oil

Method

1 Clean a dark vial thoroughly and allow it to dry.

2 Pour the ingredients into the vial, one by one.

3 Shake it well to mix the ingredients thoroughly. Be careful while shaking. Churn the vial between your palms carefully.

4 Store in a cool, dry, and dark place.

5 Has an instant relaxing effect.

Steamy Sauna Blend

Ingredients

- 25 drops juniper berry oil

- 50 drops pine oil

- 8 drops sweet birch oil

- 50 drops lemon oil

- 15 drops fir needle oil

- 8 drops wintergreen oil

Method

1   Clean a dark vial thoroughly and allow it to dry.

2   Pour the ingredients into the vial, one by one.

3   Shake it well to mix the ingredients thoroughly. Be careful while shaking. Churn the vial between your palms carefully.

4   Store in a cool, dry, and dark place.

5   Add a few drops of this concoction to a large tub with hot water and inhale the steam.

6   Cover your neck with towel for extra effect.

Soothing Lavender Skin Spray

Ingredients

- 4 ounces distilled water

- 20 drops palma rosa essential oil

- 20 drops Rose oil

- 40 drops lavender essential oil

- 10 drops sandalwood essential oil

Method

1 Clean a dark spray bottle thoroughly and allow it to dry.

2 Pour the ingredients into the vial, one by one.

3 Shake it well to mix the ingredients thoroughly. Be careful while shaking. Churn the bottle between your palms carefully. Store in a cool, dry, and dark place.

4 Spray your skin lightly for an instant fatigue relief.

Relaxing Foot Soak

Ingredients

- 20 drops Frankincense oil

- 4 drops peppermint essential oil

- 4 drops sandalwood essential oil

Method

1 Clean a dark vial thoroughly and allow it to dry.

2 Pour the ingredients into the vial, one by one.

3 Shake it well to mix the ingredients thoroughly. Be careful while shaking. Churn the vial between your palms carefully.

4 Store in a cool, dry, and dark place.

5 Add a little of the oil to a medium sized bucket of water and soak your feet in it for a refreshing and relaxing effect.

Musky Perfume Oil

Ingredients

- 15 drops cedar wood essential oil

- 24 drops Vanilla Essential oil

- 20 drops patchouli essential oil

- 20 drops frankincense essential oil

- 2 ounce Grapeseed oil

- 15 drops myrrh essential oil

Method

1 Clean a dark vial thoroughly and allow it to dry.

2 Pour the ingredients into the vial, one by one.

3 Shake it well to mix the ingredients thoroughly. Be careful while shaking. Churn the vial between your palms carefully.

4 Store in a cool, dry, and dark place.

5 Dab at pulse points for a refreshing effect.

Conclusion

I hope you would have realized the importance of aromatherapy and how it has a positive impact on your health by now. Contrary to what we think, we don't have to invest a lot of time to stay healthy. If you include the right ingredients in the right proportion, time is not an issue in the recipe for perfect health. I hope you were able to find the answers to all your questions in this book. You can also refer to the Doterra Certified Pure Therapeutic Guide for more information on essential oil uses and aromatherapy.

Try out the different recipes and see your health improving. I hope you found the book interesting. Thank you again for buying this book.

www.ingramcontent.com/pod-product-compliance
Lightning Source LLC
Chambersburg PA
CBHW060408290526
45791CB00002B/653